BEGIN THE HEALING PROCESS FROM A TOXIC TEENAGE RELATIONSHIP

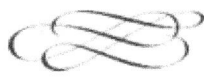

A GUIDE AND WORKBOOK OF POSITIVE AFFIRMATIONS, SELF-REFLECTION, AND JOURNAL WRITING

By

JORDAN PHOENIX, MA

Ace East Publishing LLC 1401 21st Street

Suite R

Sacramento, CA 95811

ISBN: 978-1-963939-05-7

First Edition

DISCLAIMER

This book is intended to provide educational information on the topics it covers. The author and the publisher are not providing medical, psychological, or therapeutic advice. The content of this book is not intended to be a substitute for professional medical advice, diagnosis, or treatment. Always seek the advice of your physician or other qualified health providers with any questions you may have regarding a medical condition or mental health concerns.

The stories, experiences, and advice presented in this book are based on the author's research and personal insights. They are provided as guidance and to foster understanding and empathy, not as definitive medical or psychological advice. The author and publisher disclaim any liability, loss, or risk, personal or otherwise, which is incurred as a consequence, directly or indirectly, of the use and application of any of the contents of this book.

Given the sensitive nature of the topics discussed, some content may be triggering or unsettling for young readers. Adults are encouraged to preview the material and use their discretion when sharing it with children or adolescents.

If you or someone you know is in immediate danger or needs urgent help, please contact a trusted adult, healthcare professional, or the appropriate emergency services number in your country.

For Amber & Alaina

HEALING FROM A TOXIC RELATIONSHIP

Hey there!

You've already taken an amazing journey through our main book, diving deep into understanding toxic relationships and how to heal from them. But we're not done yet – this guide is your next step to really making those changes.

Think of this guide as your personal toolbox, filled with exercises, journal prompts, and affirmations, all designed to help you apply everything you've learned. Each activity is a step forward in your healing process, from strengthening your self-esteem to building healthier relationships.

You're all set to take on something big – those unseen ties that pull us into not-so-great relationships. Yep, I've been right where you are.

Think of this not just as a book but as your new journey. A step out of the tangles of toxicity into a world where you're in charge. This isn't about blame or being stuck in yesterday. It's about getting the lowdown, healing up, and stepping forward. We can't rewind what's done, but what comes next? That's all you.

I'm here as your guide, not as some know-it-all, but as someone who's walked the walk. I've felt the whole mess of it – the hurt, the mixed-up feelings, and yeah, the awesome feeling of breaking free.

If you ever come across a term or concept that seems a bit fuzzy, don't hesitate to flip back to the main book for a quick refresher. Remember, healing is a journey, and this guide is here to support you every step of the way.

You're not alone in this, okay? Your feelings are totally legit. And there's a way through this maze. But hey, it's totally normal to feel a bit rattled or like you don't have all the answers. Recovery is more of a road trip than a quick hop. And every road trip kicks off with that first mile.

Ready to hit the road? 'Cause I totally believe in you. You've got what it takes to shake off those invisible ties and have a happier future. Let's dive in. 🚀

WHAT'S INSIDE

GASLIGHTING

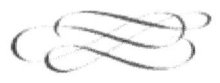

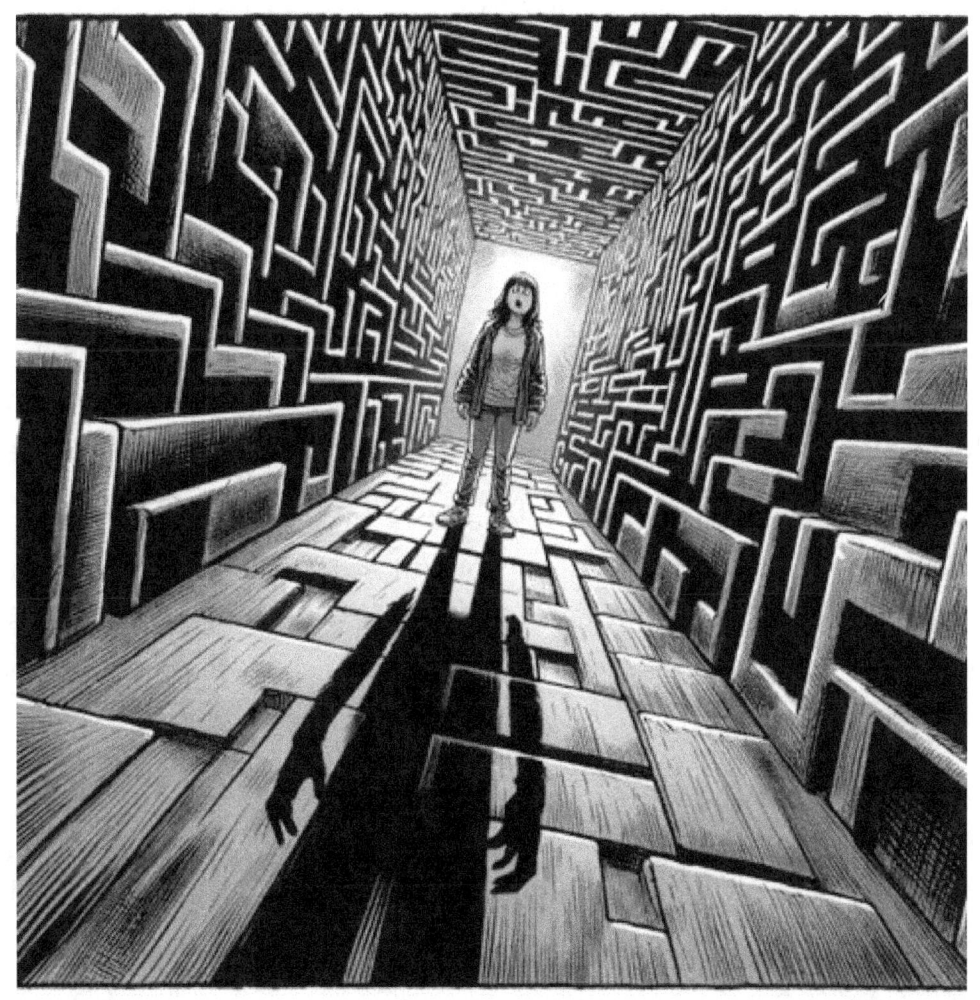

When you're being gaslit, it can feel like you're in a dark maze without any way out. You doubt your memory, thoughts, feelings, and sanity.

UN-GASLIGHTING YOURSELF

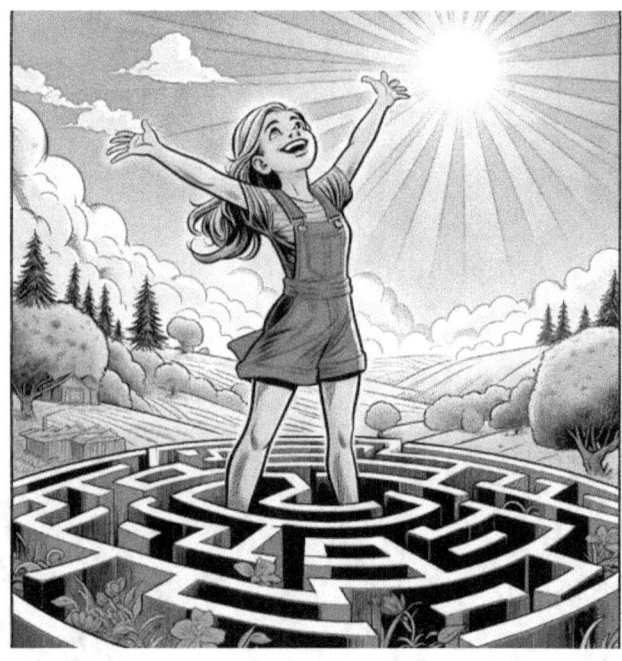

Well, guess what happens when you break free from being gaslit? It's like the maze just starts shrinking! Yep, it shrinks and shrinks until you can finally stand up tall, look around, and see the real world for what it truly is.

Becoming un-gaslit is like unlocking this epic level of freedom and self-discovery. It's about realizing the amazing person you are, away from all those fake, dark illusions your abuser threw over you like some sort of wicked spell. The moment you toss aside those bewitched black sunglasses, everything changes. You can see clearly, and suddenly, you're not under their spell anymore.

It's like you've been playing this game with a blindfold, and now it's off. You're seeing colors, lights, and paths you never knew existed. You're free from their control, free to choose your own way, and free to be the incredible person you always were under- neath their tricks. 🪄🦋

So let's take off and keep off those sunglasses. The world's a lot brighter and a lot more beautiful when you see it with your own eyes, free from anyone else's control. You've got this, and the adventure ahead is all yours! 😎🌟

MEMORY VALIDATION EXERCISE

Developing self-confidence in your own memories and thoughts can be strengthened through reflective thinking and journaling.

Here are some questions and exercises that can help you build trust in your own mind. This will help you be un-gaslit and realize your memories are valid and deserve to be considered.

Grab a piece of paper and answer these questions:

1. **Past Memory Wins**: Think about times when you remembered something spot-on, and it turned out you were totally right. What does this say about how reliable your memory can be?

2. **Your Memory Superpowers**: What stuff do you remember best? Numbers, convo details, events, faces? Realizing where you're a memory whiz can totally boost your confidence.

3. **Check Your Records**: Got old diaries, emails, or photos? See how they match up with what you remember. What does it say about your memory accuracy?

4. **Smart Decisions, Smart Thoughts**: Reflect on choices you made based on your thoughts that led to cool stuff happening. This proves your brain's on the right track!

5. **Learning from Oops Moments**: Ever realized you goofed in your thinking and then fixed it? This shows you're good at evaluating and trusting your brain.

6. **Intuition Wins**: Recall times when a gut feeling or sudden idea steered you right. These moments prove your inner guidance system is legit.

7. **Props from Your Peeps**: Remember when friends or family said, "Wow, you remembered!" or you rocked a memory game or quiz? This external high-five backs up your memory skills.

8. **Perfectly Imperfect Memory**: Everyone's memory messes up sometimes. It's totally normal, and it doesn't mean your memory is unreliable overall.

9. **How You Handle Info**: Think about how you process stuff. Do you take your time? Look at different sides of a story? This careful approach helps make your memories more accurate.

10. **Doubt vs. Evidence Showdown**: When you doubt a memory, do you look for proof or think it through logically to back it up?

11. **Chill Time with Good Memories**: Spend some time just thinking about when your memory was your superhero. How did it feel? How did it help?

12. **Consistent Thoughts**: Consider how consistent your thoughts are over time. Are your beliefs and opinions generally stable and make sense?

Building Trust with Your Brain

By diving into these exercises, you're giving your brain a high-five. You're recognizing all the cool stuff it does right, which can help shake off doubts and boost your confidence in your own thoughts and memories. Remember, your brain is like your internal Google, and it's usually pretty spot on. So trust it, and watch your self- confidence grow! 🧠👍

Keep exploring your mind's capabilities, and remember, your thoughts and memories are a big part of what makes you, you! Trust in them, and trust in yourself. You've got this! 🚀

TRUSTING YOUR MEMORY

Building trust in your own memories, mind, and feelings is essen- tial for your self-confidence and mental well-being. Here are some empowering affirmations tailored for this purpose:

1. "My memories are a valid part of my experience."

2. "I trust my memory and my ability to recall events accurately."

3. "My mind is clear, strong, and reliable."

4. "I believe in the integrity of my thoughts and feelings."

5. "Every day, my confidence in my mental abilities grows stronger."

6. "I am capable of discerning the truth in my experiences."

7. "My perceptions are grounded in reality and truth."

8. "I respect and honor my experiences and memories."

9. "I am mentally strong and independent."

10. "My thoughts and memories are an important part of who I am."

11. "I have the inner wisdom to interpret my past accurately."

12. "I am in control of my mental processes and trust in their accuracy."

13. "My mind is a powerful ally in understanding my life's journey."

14. "I embrace my experiences with clarity and confidence."

15. "Each day, my trust in my own mind becomes firmer."

16. "I am at peace with my memories and trust my interpretation of them."

17. "My feelings and memories are acknowledged and respected by me."

Using these affirmations regularly can help reinforce your belief in yourself and your mental capabilities. Whenever you feel doubtful, repeat these affirmations to remind yourself of your ability to trust your own mind and memories. It's also helpful to keep a journal of your thoughts and experiences as a way to validate and strengthen your trust in your own perceptions and memories.

YOU, ME, YES, NO, MAYBE, OH!

Who is the crazy one? They blame you, they say you can't remember stuff or are making stuff up. But who is really at fault here? Let's find out.

Answer these **6** questions to unravel the truth:

1. **Single Source Doubt**: Is it only [partner's name] who says you have a bad memory or are making things up? Think about it, do your friends or family say the same?

2. **Friends' Perspectives**: What do your friends think about your memory and perceptions? Do they ever doubt your sanity like [partner's name] does?

3. **Pre-Relationship Confidence**: Try to remember, before you met [partner's name], did you ever doubt your memory this much? If not, why do you think that's changed?

4. **Imagine a Different Scenario**: If [partner's name] never told you that you can't remember stuff or are crazy, how would you view your own memory? Would you feel differently about your sanity?

5. **Flipping the Script**: Ever considered that maybe [partner's name] is the one who's got memory issues? How would it make you feel to find out they're the forgetful one, not you?

6. **Trustworthiness Question**: Why do you think [partner's name] is more reliable with memories than you? What makes their version automatically more credible?

7. (Do not answer with "because they say so!") Could it be that they're wrong?

Flipping the Perspective: Seeing the Bigger Picture

It's super important to realize that sometimes, the issue isn't with you but with the person making you doubt yourself. These ques- tions are designed to help you see the pattern in your partner's behavior and understand that their actions might be a form of manipulation, not a reflection of your abilities.

Remember, understanding gaslighting is like solving a puzzle. It's about looking at all the pieces – your feelings, your memories, your partner's words – and seeing the real picture. Trust in your-self, your memories, and your sanity. You're smarter and stronger than you think, and you deserve to believe in yourself. 🤍🔍

VALIDATING YOUR REALITY: STAND STRONG AGAINST GASLIGHTING

Exercises to Affirm Your Perception of Reality:

1. **Recall Clear Memories**: Think of a few moments where you're 100% sure of what happened. Reflect on these memories and remind yourself how clear and certain they felt.

2. **Reaffirm What You Know**: Write down things you know to be true about yourself and your life. These could be your talents, your values, or positive moments you've experienced.

3. **Compare Perspectives**: If someone's challenging your view of an event, jot down both versions. Seeing them side by side can help you stand firm in what you know is true.

4. **Seek Objective Input**: Talk to a trusted friend or family member about an event you're unsure of. Their outside perspective can help validate your reality.

5. **Document Your Experiences**: Keep a journal of events, feelings, and reactions. Reviewing this can help reinforce your memory and perception, especially when someone tries to challenge them.

6. **Identify Gaslighting Red Flags**: Make a list of common gaslighting phrases like "You're too sensitive" or "That never happened." Recognizing these can help you stay alert to manipulation attempts.

7. **Reflect on Consistency**: Consider how consistent your memories and perceptions have been over time. This can help reinforce your trust in them.

Affirmations to Strengthen Belief in Your Reality

1. "I trust my memory and perception of events."

2. "My feelings and experiences are valid and real."

3. "I am confident in my understanding of my life and my experiences."

4. "I stand firm in my truth, even when others challenge it."

5. "I recognize and resist attempts to manipulate my perception of reality."

6. "My experiences and memories define my reality, not someone else's words."

7. "I am strong against gaslighting and trust in my inner voice."

8. "I seek truth and clarity in all situations."

9. "My perspective is valuable and deserves to be heard and respected."

10. "I am capable of discerning truth from manipulation." Embracing and Trusting Your Reality

By engaging with these exercises and repeating these affirmations, you're building a fortress of trust in your own perceptions and memories. Remember, your reality is shaped by your experiences, and you have the power to validate and trust it, no matter what others say.

Stay confident in your truth, and remember, your perspective is unique and invaluable. Trust in yourself, and you'll navigate through life's challenges with strength and clarity. You've got this!

EMOTIONAL ABUSE

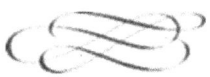

Being insulted, called names, mocked, belittled, degraded, told you're not worthy, etc... that can really ruin your self-esteem

and make you feel like you're not worthy of anything good. Know that those are just negative echoes from the abuse you suffered, NOT the truth. In this chapter, we'll help you get rid of those fake beliefs and increase your self-worth.

WORTHY, NOT WORTHY... WHICH IS TRUE?

When Insults Start to Sound Like 'Truth'

Ever notice how, when someone keeps dissing you, you start to wonder if they're onto something? You might think, "If they keep saying I'm [insert mean comment here], maybe it's true?"

But here's the deal: just because someone says something doesn't make it your reality. 🚫

Their Words vs. Your Reality

Picture this: You're in an art gallery, right? There's this wild painting on the wall, all abstract and stuff. Three peeps are standing there, checking it out.

Person 1: "OMG, this is the most beautiful thing ever!"

Person 2: "Yuck, this is the ugliest painting I've ever seen!"

Person 3: "Meh, it's alright, kinda in the middle for me."

So, who's right? What's the 'truth' here?

Spoiler: There's no one 'truth' – it's all about perspective!

That painting isn't changing – it's the same bunch of colors and strokes. But to one person, it's a masterpiece; to another, it's a disaster; and to someone else, it's just meh. Their opinions don't change what the painting actually is; they're just different views.

Your Worth Isn't Defined by Their Opinion

Here's how this painting thing ties into real life. Let's talk about Judy. She's super skinny, and her first BF was all about trying to 'fatten her up.' He'd be like, "You're too skinny, you're all bones. I hate skinny girls!" Judy felt terrible, thinking she was ugly and unlovable.

But plot twist: They break up, and she meets Drew, who's totally into skinny girls. He's all, "You're gorgeous! I love your thin wrists, your ankles, everything!" For Drew, skinny is his type.

See, Judy didn't change – she's still the same person. But the opin- ions about her did. What her ex thought of her body was his deal, not hers. His words didn't define her beauty or worth; they were just his opinion, based on his likes and dislikes.

Questions to Get You Thinking

Q1: The Skinny on Worthiness

So, Judy's skinny – does that make her any less worthy of love? Think about it. Does her waist size have a VIP pass to her heart?

Q2: Change for Love – Yay or Nay?

Do you really think Judy needs to change herself to be loved? Is it about swapping her jeans size or finding someone who digs her style as is?

Q3: Makeover Time – Herself or Her Circle?

What's the real change needed for Judy – a new look or a new crew? Should she be flipping through fashion mags or flipping the script on who she hangs with?

Real Talk on Change

Who's Got the Issue? Spoiler: Not Judy

The problem isn't with Judy or her body; it's about being with someone who's not vibing with her as she is. You can't remix other people's tastes, but you can totally choose who you share your playlist with.

If someone's throwing shade your way, if they're not loving the awesome you, maybe it's not about a personal rebrand. Maybe it's about finding peeps who celebrate your brand of awesome. Trust me, they're out there!

The Affirmation You Gotta Repeat

"What they say about me is just their opinion. It's not the truth about who I am. Their words and what they think are totally not the same as my worth. I'm like this gem with my own sparkle, and that doesn't change with someone else's weather report.

I'm 100% lovable just as I am. No edits needed."

Remember, you're not a rough draft needing edits; you're a final print, perfect in your own story. Stay true to your plot – it's worth the read! 📖💜

" WHY' S MY PARTNER ACTING LIKE A MONSTER?"

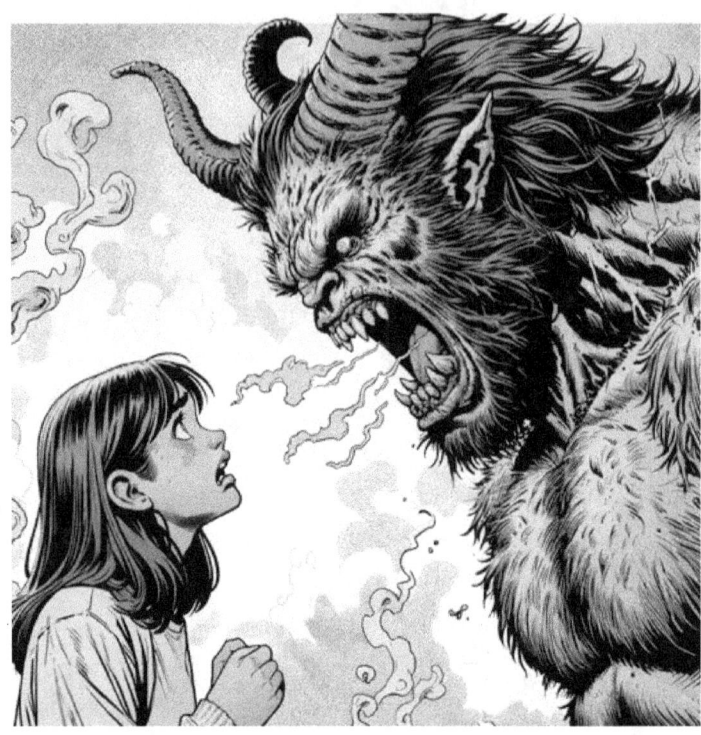

Ever wonder, "Why would my BF/GF want to hurt me?" Okay, so here's the thing: psychology is like this huge, complicated puzzle. Some peeps, including those who turn out to be not-so-great partners, have been through tough stuff themselves. They're carrying around this hurt, like thorns poking them from the inside. Ouch, right?

Sometimes, they don't know how to deal with these 'thorns,' so they lash out. Imagine that each time they get toxic or abusive, they're turning into this 'ugly monster.' This monster? It's not about them being evil; it's like a messed-up symbol of the pain and problems they haven't dealt with.

But here's the real talk: Their issues and their monster-like moments? They're not about you. They don't show your value; they show their struggles.

No Excuses for Being Cruel

And hey, important side note: Even if they've had a rough past, it's never, ever an excuse to treat you badly. You deserve respect and kindness, period. No buts or becauses – just straight-up love and respect.

MIRROR, MIRROR, NOT SO CLEAR: WHY THEY SAY HURTFUL STUFF

Okay, think about a mirror. Normally, it shows exactly what's in front of it. But if that mirror's all twisted or cracked, things get wonky. Like, imagine a tall, thin girl looking in this funky mirror and seeing herself all wavy and weird. That's not her; that's the mirror messing up the reflection.

That's kind of like what's going on with someone who's abusive. Their view of the world, and you, is like looking through a busted mirror. Their words and actions? They're coming from this distorted place filled with their own probs and insecurities.

So, when they say something hurtful, remember, it's like that wonky mirror. It's not showing you as you are; it's showing their messed-up version of reality.

You're Not Their Words

What they say, how they see you – that's on them, not you. Your worth, your smarts, your beauty – they're shining bright, no matter what they're spitting out. You're not the reflection in their cracked mirror; you're the real deal, all by yourself.

AFFIRMATIONS TO KEEP YOU GROUNDED

Affirmations are like spells; they're magic little sentences that help you feel better and increase your self-confidence. Simply repeat them multiple times out loud whenever you feel confused, hurt, unloved, and unsure about yourself.

"I'm in charge of my actions, not theirs."

"I'm not the reason for someone else's mean streak." "When they're mean, it's because they have a problem. It's not because of me."

"It's not my fault someone is mean to me. It's their choices, their mess. Not mine."

Remember, you're your own person, not someone's shadow or a character in their messed-up story. Keep shining your light, and don't let anyone's inner monster dim it. You got this! 💪🖤

POSITIVITY EXERCISE: YOU VS. THEIR WORDS

Okay, so let's do a little exercise to help put some space between you and those hurtful words.

Step 1: Their Words on Paper

Grab a piece of paper and write down some of the stuff that's been said to you. Seeing it outside of your head can make a big difference.

Step 2: Who You Really Are

Now, on another piece of paper, write down all the amazing things about you. Your talents, your dreams, the compliments you've received, moments when you felt proud of yourself. Think of nice little things and big things that make you special.

This is the real you.

Step 3: Compare and Contrast

Hold those two pieces of paper side by side. See how different they are? That's because what people say about you doesn't define you. You're defined by your own strengths, achievements, and the love you carry in your heart. 🩶

Step 4: Trash Talk

Now, if you're feeling it, crumple up the first piece of paper – the one with the insults – and toss it in the trash. That's where it belongs. Not in your mind, not in your heart.

REFRAME IT!

Here's how to flip the script. Every time you catch yourself feeling down from an insult, pause. Ask yourself, 'What's something nice about me?' Remember, you're awesome, smart, funny... whatever makes you, you. 👣 Start to see yourself through that lens of posi- tivity, not through the negativity others throw at you.

AFFIRMATION REPL ACEMENT EXERCISE

Step 1: Uncover Your Negative Beliefs

First, let's find out what negative beliefs might be lurking in your mind. Fill in the blanks in these questions to reveal them. Think about what you often feel or have been made to believe in your relationship:

1. "I'm not _____enough." (smart, good, pretty, etc.)

2. "I'm _____worthy of love." (un, not)

3. "I always _____" (mess up, fail, etc.)

4. "I don't deserve _____" (happiness, success, love)

5. "I'm too _____ to be loved." (flawed, different, etc.)

Write down these negative beliefs. Seeing them on paper can be powerful and eye-opening.

Step 2: Create Your Positive Affirmations

Now, for each negative belief you've written, let's flip it to create a positive affirmation. This is where you take back your power. Here's how you can transform them:

1. If you wrote, "I'm not smart enough," change it to: "**I am intelligent in my own unique way.**"

2. For "I'm unworthy of love," it becomes: "**I am worthy of love and respect.**"

3. If it's "I always mess up," turn it into: "**I learn and grow from every experience.**"

4. Change "I don't deserve happiness" to: "**I deserve happiness and joy in my life.**"

5. If you wrote, "I'm too flawed to be loved," it becomes: "**My flaws are part of my unique beauty, and I am lovable as I am.**"

Write these affirmations down as your new truths.

Step 3: Repeat Your Positive Affirmations

Now, repeat these positive affirmations to yourself. Do it every day, multiple times a day. Say them out loud, write them in your journal, put them on sticky notes around your room – whatever works for you.

- "I am intelligent in my own unique way."

- "I am worthy of love and respect."

- "I learn and grow from every experience."

- "I deserve happiness and joy in my life."

- "My flaws are part of my unique beauty, and I am lovable as I am."

Remember: You Are in Control

By repeating these affirmations, you're rewiring your brain to believe in your worth and value. You're taking control of your story, your self-view. It's a powerful way to heal and grow stronger.

You're not the negative things you've been made to believe. You're so much more. Keep using these affirmations to remind yourself of your true worth. You're amazing, just as you are! 💜

Positive Affirmations Are like Your Secret Superpower

Your brain is like this super-smart computer. ▪ And what you feed it makes a huge difference in how you feel and see the world.

When you repeat positive affirmations, it's like you're program- ming your brain to focus on the good stuff. It helps shift your mindset from "I can't" to "I totally got this." It's not magic, but it sure feels like it sometimes.

Write 'Em, Say 'Em, Believe 'Em

Grab a pen and some paper and write down some positive affir- mations. They can be from the list we made or ones you come up with yourself. The key? They should be about how awesome, capa- ble, and loved you are.

Then, make it a habit. Every morning, or whenever you need a pick-me-up, say these affirmations out loud. Look in the mirror and tell yourself these truths. It might feel weird at first, but give it time. You're planting seeds of positivity that will totally bloom.

Watch the Magic Happen

Over time, you'll start to notice a change. Those downer thoughts get a little quieter, and the positive ones start taking center stage. You'll feel more confident, more you. And that's when you realize: You've got the power to shape your world, one affirmation at a time.

POSITIVE AFFIRMATIONS

Whenever you feel down, repeat these positive affirmations out loud and write them down. You'll be amazed at how good it feels!

1. "I am worthy of respect and kindness."

2. "What someone says does not define me."

3. "My worth is not defined by their words."

4. "I am more than enough just as I am."

5. "I deserve a relationship that makes me feel good about myself."

6. "I am strong enough to stand up against negativity."

7. "My feelings and experiences are valid."

8. "I am capable of creating positive change in my life."

9. "I can achieve anything I want."

10. "I have inner value."

11. "I am good enough."

12. "I am valuable."

Affirmations are powerful and can totally transform your outlook. Keep those positive vibes flowing, and remember, you're the boss of your own thoughts. Rock on!

DEBUNKING NEGATIVE BELIEFS

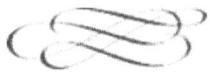

YOU MATTER, AND I MATTER: THE TALE OF TWO APPLES

The Story of Big Red and Little Green

Imagine a tree, like the one you might chill under at the park. It's got loads of apples, each getting life-giving tree sap. They're all thriving, doing their apple thing.

But here's the drama: There's this one apple, let's call him Big Red. He's kinda the big shot of the branch. He's full of himself and feels really important.

One day, he's like, "Yo, I want ALL the sap, because I'm the MVP here. I matter more than all of you."

Next to him is this smaller, kinda shy apple, Little Green. He tries to speak up, but Big Red just shuts him down. "You? You don't matter, dude! It's all about what I want! Hand over your sap!"

Little Green gets all intimidated, feeling small and like he doesn't count. So, he lets Big Red take all his sap. Big Red gets bigger and shinier, while Little Green? He's just withering away, getting all shriveled and sad. Falling apart, starving to death...

What's Fair, What's Not

So, let's think about this. Is this fair? Does Big Red really deserve all the sap? What about Little Green? Doesn't he have a right to that life-giving sap too?

Little Green's over here thinking, "I guess I don't deserve the sap. Big Red said so. He's the important one, right? I just gave him what he wanted 'cause my needs don't matter."

Your Turn to Speak Up

Now, it's your turn to drop some truth bombs. What would you say to Little Green? How would you convince him that he matters just as much as Big Red?

Tell Little Green what you think:_____

Wrapping Up: Every Apple Deserves Sap

In the story of Big Red and Little Green, it's clear that every apple on that tree deserves its share of sap. Just like in life, everyone – including you – deserves respect, care, and the chance to thrive. 🌳

No one person's wants are more important than another person's wants. You matter just as much as your partner or anyone else.

You are just as worthy of love, respect, happiness, and all the good things you want as anyone else!

EMPOWERING AFFIRMATIONS

To strengthen yourself and be able to resist manipulation, it's important to realize that your opinions are just as valid as anyone else's. What you want matters just as much as what someone else wants.

Why should one person's wants be more important than another person's?

Why should their wants override someone else's?

To increase your self-confidence and not let others manipulate you anymore, repeat these affirmations often:

What one person says about me does not define what I am. I have inner value and worth no matter what someone says.

What they say doesn't define what I am. I am a great person always.

I am fully worthy of being treated with love and respect. My opinions are real, they matter, they are valid.

It's okay for me to have my own opinions. My opinions matter.

It's okay for me to do what I want. My wants and needs matter.

I matter.

I am important. I am valuable.

My feelings are just as important as [partner's name]. My opinions are just as valid as [partner's name].

I am just as important as [partner's name]. I matter just as much as anyone else.

Being unique is great. I don't need to be a copy of anyone else.

I am worthy of love even if I'm unique and different from anyone else.

"A M I WORTHY OF LOVE OR NOT?"

Jane's Wild Walk with the "Worthiness Meter"

Picture this: Jane's strutting down the street, and she's got this funky digital "worthiness meter" hovering over her head. And get this – she set it so ANYONE and everyone can mess with it. Why? 'Cause she thinks maybe they know her worth better than she does.

As she's walking, people are shouting their judgments at her, based on what? Their own likes and dislikes. One person's "NOT WORTHY," just 'cause they're not feeling her skirt. Another's like, "TOTALLY WORTHY," loving the same skirt. Then someone disses her for being blonde, and another boosts her score for it. Talk about confusing, right? Her meter's going nuts, flipping from green to red, up and down. Jane's feeling all kinds of mixed ups and downs – happy one moment and sad the next.

So, think about this wild scene. Can these random opinions about her look really say if Jane's a good person or not? They don't even know her! They're just shouting based on a quick glance.

Who Should Control the Meter?

Why should Jane let her worth be tossed around by other people's random and clashing views? Imagine if she just set that meter to "worthy" herself and didn't let anyone else mess with it. Do you think she'd feel better, more chill, knowing her worth's not up for public debate?

And here's another thing: Why should someone get treated better just 'cause they fit someone else's idea of pretty, smart, or cool? That doesn't make sense, right?

So, Jane's story? It's like a big, flashing neon sign saying, "You define your worth, not anyone else."

Keep your meter set to "worthy," 'cause guess what?

You totally are, no matter what anyone else shouts from the sidelines. 🚀

Self-Worth and Love: The Real Deal

Everyone's worthy of love, no exceptions!

Yo, remember this: Every single person is totally worthy of love, no matter how they look. Nobody's opinion has the power to decide if you're lovable or not. 🚫🩶

Think about it: People dig different things. One person might be all about ginger cats, while another is team white cat all the way. What one person's not into, someone else might totally adore.

And get this: Even peeps who've made big mistakes or seem 'unworthy' (like criminals or those history book villains) can find love. It's all about realizing that one person's view doesn't define how lovable you are.

Love isn't a perfection contest.

Love's not about hitting some high score on a 'perfect partner' scale. It's about finding someone who gets you, loves you for you – quirks, curves, and all.

" I FEEL I ' M NOT GOOD ENOUGH THE WAY I AM"

So, picture this: You're in this beautiful flower garden, right? And each flower in this garden is like a person in the world. Some flowers pop open super early, while others take their sweet time. You've got tall flowers, short ones, some rocking bright colors, and others with chill, low-key vibes. Each flower, just by being itself, makes the garden this amazing, diverse place.

Now, think about you as one of these flowers. Just by being you – with your own style, your own pace, and your own color – you're adding something special to the world's garden.

This garden? It's a lot like humanity. Each person, including you, is enough just by being themselves. You don't need to be taller, brighter, or anything else – you're perfect for your spot in the garden, adding your own unique kind of awesome.

In humanity's garden, everyone fits in.

ROLE-PL AY GAME: HELPING EMMA FEEL LOVED

Imagine you have a friend called Emma. She's super sweet, always there for you, great at keeping secrets, encourages you and makes you feel really happy. Like a really great friend. But now this guy she's into called her a 'fat cow,' and now she's feeling like no one will ever love her. She says, "I'm too overweight to be loved."

Your mission? Lift her spirits with some truth bombs about love and worth.

Questions to Ponder and How to Reply

1. Can One Person Decide Emma's Lovability?

Your Reply: _____

Jane's Reply: No way! Everyone's got their own taste. Just 'cause one dude's not into her doesn't mean someone else won't think she's amazing.

2. Why Could Emma Still Find Love?

Your Reply: _____

Jane's Reply: There are so many peeps out there, and someone's bound to dig Emma just as she is. Plus, she's a super nice person.

3. What Rocks About Emma's Friendship?

Your Reply: _____

Jane's Reply: Her personality, for sure! She's the kind of friend who makes life brighter, no matter what she looks like.

4. Team Emma or Team Lara?

Lara is this really beautiful skinny girl. But her personality is like a snake covered in thorns. She's all about finding faults, insulting people, and sharing their secrets to hurt them.

So, whom would you rather be friends with? Beauty queen Lara or kind Emma?

Your Reply: _____

Jane's Reply: 100% Team Emma. Being nice and real matters way more than just looks.

5. Could a BF Dig Emma's Awesome Traits?

Your Reply: _____

Jane's Reply: Emma, you're totally lovable! You're this amazing person who deserves all the love.

Boosting Emma's Confidence

Emma: "I'm not worthy of love."

You: _____

By reflecting on Emma's situation, we get to see how our own views on worth and love shape our world. It's about understanding that worthiness isn't skin deep – it's about who we are on the inside. 🖤🪶

BELIEF CHECK: " I FEEL LIKE EVERYTHING' S ALWAYS MY FAULT!"

Imagine you're part of a dance duo. It's all about moving together, right? But let's say your dance partner steps on your toes. Ouch! And then they blame you!

Is it only your fault for having your toes stepped on? Doesn't quite sound fair, does it? They stepped on you, and then they're blaming you!

In the 'dance' of a relationship, both partners play their parts. If something goes offbeat, it's not just on one person. Blaming your- self all the time? That's like saying you're responsible for every misstep, even the ones you didn't make.

In the dance of relationships, it's about teamwork, not solo guilt trips.

If someone's trying to blame it all on you every time, that's toxic, and you totally don't have to accept it.

Just because someone says it's your fault doesn't mean it actually is!

BUILDING YOUR TREASURE TROVE

The best way to feel better about yourself is to remember all the little things that make you awesome. Take out a journal or note- book and write answers to these questions:

1. When was a time you felt really good about yourself? Describe it.

2. List 3 good things about yourself. It could be your hair, your nose, or some positive parts of your personality.

3. List 5 times you did something really well. It could be an exam you aced, a contest you won, a new hobby you mastered, or a great idea you got. Something that made you feel happy, proud, special, smart, cool, or unique. For instance, Jane remembers having climbed a very high wall. Liz remembers the first time she managed to ride a horse. Ron remembers how awesome it felt to learn to ski and rocket down the mountainside faster than all his friends.

4. Beneath your 5 good memories, write down what that means about you. For instance, if you overcame something really difficult, that means you're resilient, strong, and a

winner. To figure out what it means about you, think "winning the game means I am...". Your answer could be "a winner, strong, capable, driven, focused, a great player..."

Then phrase it as an affirmation: "I am a winner." "I am capable." "I am strong." "People like me." Stuff like that.

The next time someone tells you that you're a loser, remember the time you succeeded and tell yourself "I am a winner, and I can win again."

GUILT TRIPS

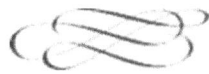

Aguilt trip is when someone makes you feel guilty for not doing what they want. For instance, they might say you're

selfish for doing the things you want, like hanging out with friends instead of being there for them all the time. The truth is this is just a cheap manipulation. To not let them drag you along on their fake guilt trip, here are some affirmations to help you strengthen your self-esteem and self-respect.

AFFIRMATIONS TO COUNTER GUILT TRIPS

- I have the right to my own time and space.

- Choosing for myself doesn't make me selfish or ungrateful.

- I am not responsible for others' happiness.

- My feelings and needs are just as important as anyone else's.

- Saying 'no' does not make me a bad person or partner.

- I deserve to pursue my own interests and hobbies.

- I am worthy of respect and understanding.

- My value isn't measured by how much I sacrifice for others.

- I choose to act out of love, not guilt.

- I am strong enough to resist manipulation and stand by my choices.

- It's okay for me to do the things I want, just like it's okay for others to do what they want.

- I let others live their lives the way they want. And I deserve to be treated the same way.

- It's okay for me to have my own life and to live it the way that I want.

JOURNAL PROMPT EXERCISE TO RECL AIM YOUR POWER

Reflect on these questions:

1. Think of a time you felt guilt-tripped. What was the situation? How did you react?

2. What are some things you enjoy doing for yourself that others have made you feel guilty about? Write down why it's totally okay for you to do those things and why you're still a good person.

3. How do you feel when you do things out of guilt? (Spoiler: Any time you feel bad, that's a sign of something being seriously off. It's like an inner compass that's screaming "TOXIC!")

4. Reflect on how you can balance your own needs with your relationships.

5. Remind yourself daily that your needs and wants are valid. Start with "My wants and needs..."

AFFIRMATIONS TO CL AIM YOUR INDEPENDENCE

Remember, you're an awesome original, not a copy. These affirma- tions are here to remind you of that. Say them, believe them, live them!

1. **"My style is my signature."**

- Rock those clothes, that hair, that look. It's your style, and it's amazing.

2. **"My hobbies and passions are my playground."**

- Whether it's gaming, painting, or playing guitar, your hobbies are all about you being you.

3. **" My feelings are valid, always."**

- Happy, sad, excited, or mad – your feelings are real and totally yours.

4. **" My thoughts are my power."**

- Your ideas and opinions? They're valuable and worth sharing.

5. **" My wants and needs matter."**

- What you want and need is important – from the food you love to the dreams you chase.

6. **" I am in charge of my happiness."**

- Your joy is yours to create and cherish, no one else's.

7. **" My voice is unique and deserves to be heard."**

- Speak up, speak out. Your voice adds to the world's melody.

8. **" I am the author of my story. I am in control of my life. I am in control of my future."**

- Write your chapters and choose your adventures. It's your life story.

9. **"I am enough, just as I am."**

- No 'ifs,' 'buts,' or 'shoulds.' You're perfectly you, and that's more than enough.

10. **"I choose my path and walk it with confidence."**

- Your journey, your steps. Walk them with your head held high.

Every time you feel like someone's trying to dim your shine or change your tune, remember these affirmations and say them to yourself (even quietly). You're the boss of your world, your choices, your life. Don't let anyone tell you otherwise. You're a star, and stars are meant to shine bright, in their own way.

So, go out there and be unapologetically you. Your independence – your uniqueness – is your superpower. Embrace it, celebrate it, and own it. You got this!

JOURNALING EXERCISE: CELEBRATE UNIQUENESS

Exploring the Fame of Being Unique

1. **Pick 3 Celebs with a Unique Vibe**: Think of three famous people who totally stand out because of their style, talents, music, or even their looks. Jot them down.

2. **How Did Their Uniqueness Rock Their World?** Write about how their unique qualities helped them become rich, famous, loved, or popular. Did their one-of-a-kind style make them a household name? Did their unusual talent skyrocket them to fame?

Deep Dive Questions:

- **Q1) What If They Were 'Normal'?** Imagine if these celebs had ditched their uniqueness and gone for a regular life. Like, what if Rihanna had become a secretary instead of a music icon? How different would her life be? Would she still be the beloved star she is today?

- **Q2) Why Being Unique is Awesome**: Why do you think being different is a good thing? What makes standing out from the crowd something to celebrate?

- **Q3) What are some benefits of being unique?** What 'good' can come out of it? List 3 positive things that happened to unique people.

Recognizing Your Own Unique Superpowers:

Now, think about what makes YOU special. Write down three things that make you uniquely awesome. Maybe it's your chill vibe, a hidden talent, or your quirky sense of style.

Try continuing these sentences:

"I have a unique..." "My... is unique..." "I have a great..."

Turning 'Flaws' into Wins:

Next, list three things you think are 'not-so-great' unique traits about yourself. Now, flip the script! How can these traits be seen as positives? Like, if you have super sensitive hearing, your friends might give you a hard time and maybe you feel bad because you can't attend loud rock concerts. But hey, those ears are unique! Maybe you're a natural for a career in music production or sound engineering.

How do your unique traits help you right now? Maybe your keen hearing lets you enjoy music on a deeper level or makes you the family's official "car-approaching" alert system.

Get creative and think of some wild, fun ways your uniqueness could shape your future. Could your love for detailed doodling make you a sought-after graphic designer? Your knack for remem- bering random facts make you a quiz show champ?

Wrapping Up: Embracing Your Uniqueness

Your uniqueness is your superpower, and this exercise is all about embracing it. Whether it's something that makes you stand out or a trait you're learning to love, it's all part of what makes you, well, you! So keep celebrating your unique self, and who knows where your special qualities will take you!

Remember, in the grand story of life, your uniqueness is your signature. It's what makes your chapter so exciting and unforget- table. Keep writing your story, one unique trait at a time. You're amazing just the way you are!

JOURNALING EXERCISE: 3 GOOD THINGS ABOUT YOU

Write down 3 special unique things about yourself. These could be your kind personality, a special skill or a talent, or even just how you look. Remember, some people became famous and rich just because of their looks – including 'unusual' looks.

Be a Hero in Someone's Story - Spread Kindness Like Confetti

"Kindness is a language which the deaf can hear and the blind can see."

— **MARK TWAIN**

Ever heard the saying, "What goes around, comes around"? Well, it's time to sprinkle some kindness and watch it grow into some- thing beautiful. Here's a little secret: doing good for others doesn't just help them; it gives you a happiness boost, too!

Now, I've got a tiny but mighty favor to ask you...

Would you be willing to light up someone's world, someone you might not even know? Imagine them a bit like your younger self: eager to grow, hoping for change, and searching for a guiding light but not quite sure where to find it.

Our hearts and soul are poured into making recovery from toxic relationships a beacon of hope for everyone. Our dream? To spread this message far and wide. But we've got a small challenge: reaching every single person who needs this guide.

And here's where you, yes YOU, come in. Believe it or not, your voice is powerful. A lot of folks decide on a book based on what others say about it. So, on behalf of a teen navigating through a toxic relationships somewhere out there:

<u>Your mission, should you choose to accept, is to share your thoughts on this book.</u>

This isn't about spending money. It's about donating a few moments of your time, which could forever alter the course of another teen's life. Your review has the magic to:

...help one more person feel understood and less alone.

...support someone in finding the courage to seek healthier rela- tionships.

...offer a lifeline to those drowning in doubt and confusion.

...inspire another soul to reclaim their confidence and happiness.

...turn someone's life story from despair to hope.

Feeling that warm glow inside already? To make your act of kind- ness a reality (in under a minute!), here's what to do:

leave a heartfelt review.

Just zap the QR code right here:

[https://www.amazon.com/review/review-your-purchases/? asin=BOOKASIN]

If the thought of helping a struggling teen out there makes your heart happy, you're definitely our kind of superhero. Welcome to the squad!

I'm super thrilled to embark on this journey with you toward a Toxic-Free Life with more confidence than you ever imagined. You're gonna be wowed by the guidance and insight waiting for you in the chapters ahead.

A million thanks for being awesome. Let's dive back into trans- forming lives together.

LEAVE A REVIEW!

- Your cheerleader,

Jordan Phoenix

LIES AND MANIPULATIONS

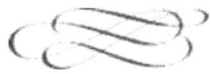

UNRAVELING THE DANGEROUS WEB OF ' FALSE TRUTHS'

Ever notice how, sometimes, a small bit of truth gets twisted into a big, hurtful lie? That's what we call 'false truths.' It's like someone takes one tiny thing and blows it up into a full-on attack on who you are.

How They Generalize and Hurt

The Ugly Hairdo Becomes "You're Ugly": Say you try a new hairdo, and someone doesn't like it. Instead of just dissing the hairstyle, they go all, "You look ugly." Bam! Suddenly, it's not about the hair; it's about you as a person. **One Lost Game Turns Into "You're a Loser"**: You lose a sports match, and someone's like, "You're such a loser." Ouch. It's not just the game you lost; now it feels like your whole identity is being called a 'loser.'

The Harmful Impact

These kinds of insults can really mess with your head. You start thinking, "Am I really a failure or ugly?" Your self-esteem takes a hit, and your confidence? Down the drain. It's like wearing glasses that make everything about you look bad.

Sometimes, in a relationship, one person tries to play this twisted game where they use 'false truths' to make you feel small. Let's talk about Derek and his GF as an example.

Derek's Story: The Eiffel Tower Trap

Derek's GF is like a walking trivia game. She knows all sorts of random facts, like how fast a llama can sprint or the number of stairs in the Eiffel Tower. Cool, right? But here's the catch: She uses this knowledge to put Derek down. When Derek can't answer her trivia questions, she's all, "You don't know how many stairs the Eiffel Tower has? You're a stupid idiot! You don't know anything!"

The Half-Truth Hook

See, she's hooking him with a half-truth. Yeah, Derek doesn't know some random fact, but does that make him stupid? Heck no! But because there's a tiny bit of truth in what she says (the part about not knowing the number of stairs), Derek starts to believe the whole thing, including the 'stupid idiot' part.

Breaking Down the 'False Truth' Technique

This is where we need to get our detective hats on and do some critical thinking. Just because one part of a statement is true doesn't make the whole thing true. It's like a sandwich with a slice of truth and a whole lot of nonsense.

Critical Thinking to the Rescue

So, here's how to break it down:

Acknowledge the Fact: "Okay, so I don't know the number of stairs. True."

Challenge the Insult: "But hey, not knowing that doesn't make me stupid. I know tons of other cool stuff!"

Remember, your intelligence isn't measured by trivia, not knowing something someone asks, or measuring yourself against others. It's about how you think, learn, and see the world. Not knowing one thing doesn't erase all the awesome stuff you do know.

Flipping the Script: Own Your Knowledge

The next time someone tries to pull a 'Derek's GF' on you, remem- ber: what you don't know doesn't define you. You're smart in your own way, and not knowing one thing doesn't change who you are.

By understanding the trick of 'false truths,' you can start to see when someone's trying to manipulate you with half-baked state- ments. Stick to your guns, and remember, your worth isn't a quiz score. You're way more than that. Stay sharp, stay you!

Beliefs Shaping Actions

Our beliefs drive what we do and how we react. When you start buying into these false truths, like thinking you're unworthy or not good enough, it can change the whole course of your life. You might hold back from going after what you want, feel like you don't deserve good stuff, or worse, believe you deserve the bad stuff.

The Example of Jenny

Take Jenny, for example. She failed an exam, and someone told her, "You're so stupid." Since 'being stupid' seemed like a 'logical' reason, she believed it. Now, she's scared to speak up, try new things, or chase her dreams. It's like one false belief put up a bunch of roadblocks in her life.

Abusers' Manipulative Tactics

Abusers are pros at this game. They use these false truths to make their victims feel small, unworthy, and at fault. It's a way to keep control. If you believe you're the problem, you're less likely to stand up for yourself or think you deserve better.

It's the main reason why people let their partner hurt them, insult them, hit them, and even sexually abuse them – because they think they deserve it!

The Danger of Accepting False Truths

These false truths, because they seem to make sense at first, can trap you in a cycle of negative thinking. You start accepting the abuse, blaming yourself, feeling guilty, and thinking you're not worthy of anything better. It's like living in a world where every mirror shows a distorted version of you.

But here's the thing: Just because someone says it doesn't make it true. You're not what they say you are. You're way more than a failed test, a lost game, or a hairstyle. You're a whole person with a ton of worth, and no one's flawed opinion can change that. 🩶

Remember, you have the power to challenge these false truths. Don't let someone else's words dictate your worth. You're worthy, you're enough, and you definitely deserve a life filled with love and respect. Stay strong and trust in your own truth. 🚀

EXAMPLES

The "Always Wrong" Trap

Alex and Sam are chillin' together, and Sam's talking about her favorite band. Out of nowhere, Alex goes, "You got the song title wrong. You always get things wrong." Sam starts to feel like maybe she's not that smart after all.

Typical Sentence: "You're always messing up. Can't you get anything right?"

The "Never Good Enough" Game

Bella tries her best to look nice for her date with Jordan. But when she shows up, Jordan smirks, "You're wearing that? You never look as good as other girls." Bella's confidence starts to crumble, feeling she'll never be pretty enough.

Typical Sentence: "Why can't you look more like [insert name]? You never dress well."

The "Constant Comparison" Con

Every time Mike and his GF, Leah, hang out, she compares him to her ex, saying things like, "My ex would have known how to fix this. You're just clueless." Mike begins to doubt his abilities, feeling inferior.

Typical Sentence: "My ex was so much better at this than you. You just don't measure up."

The "Love With Conditions" Lie

Emma's BF, Tyler, often says, "If you really loved me, you'd do this for me." So, Emma bends over backward, trying to prove her love, fearing that she's not loving enough as she is.

Typical Sentence: "If you really loved me, you wouldn't argue. You'd just do what I say."

The "Isolation Tactic" Twist

Whenever Hannah wants to hang with friends, her BF, Chris, guilts her, saying, "You'd rather be with them than me. Guess I'm not important." Hannah starts to feel guilty for having a life outside of him.

Typical Sentence: "You always choose others over me. I guess I'm just not that important to you."

Remember, these 'false truths' are nothing more than manipula- tion tactics. They're designed to make you doubt yourself and feel reliant on the abuser. It's important to recognize them for what they are – tools of control, not reflections of your true worth. You're way more than these twisted words. Stay aware and stay strong!

EVIL BRAIN TRICKS DECODED

Did you know that those sneaky manipulative tricks, the 'false truths,' are super common in not-so-great relationships? So common, in fact, that experts have studied them and given them fancy names! It's like they're the go-to weapons for people looking to control or put others down.

When someone's throwing these false truths at you, remember, it's not you that's the problem. It's them using these well-known, manipulative strategies. They're like relationship clichés, used by people all over the world to play mind games.

Now let's dive into some high-level stuff. We're talking about some university-level brain gymnastics here, so if you get this, you're basically a genius! 🚀

We're about to expose 'false truths' (or as experts call them, 'logical fallacies') used in manipulative relationships.

Understanding these is like having a secret decoder for when someone's trying to mess with you. It will help you see clearly when something is NOT true so you don't fall for these fake truths. Trust me, it will save you a lot of heartache.

Next time someone tries to hit you with one of these, you can totally flip the script. Imagine them saying something mean, and you spin around, all cool and collected, and hit them with, "Nice try, but that's just an 'Ad Hominem' fallacy. You're trying to make me feel bad and control me. Not cool. I'm not [whatever they said]." Watch their jaws drop when you call out their game with those fancy terms. It's like having a secret superpower in the world of words. 📚✨

So, now you're not just defending yourself; you're schooling them in psychology and logic. How awesome is that? Keep this knowl- edge in your back pocket, and remember, you're way smarter than their mind tricks. 🎓🖤

The List of 'False Truths' (aka Fallacies) Used to Manipulate and Control:

1. The 'You're Just...' Attack (Ad Hominem Fallacy):

- When they attack you instead of the topic or problem. Like, "You're just too stupid to get what I mean." "You're too young to understand" "You're a boy, of course you wouldn't get it."

2. The 'If You Loved Me' Trick (Emotional Appeal Fallacy):

- Emotional blackmail alert! "If you really loved me, you wouldn't do what I want."

- Love doesn't have conditions. You can show your love in many ways. You don't have to do XYZ to prove your love.

3. **The 'You're Saying I...' Misfire** (Straw Man Fallacy):

- Twisting your words. "You want some alone time? So, you're saying you don't want to be with me?"

- Wanting time alone is one thing, not wanting to be with you is completely separate. Twisting them together is manipulation (trying to get you to not spend any time alone but just be together all the time).

4. **The 'One Thing Leads to Disaster' Slide** (Slippery Slope Fallacy):

- Overreacting to small things and thinking one little thing will lead to a bigger thing. "Going out with friends tonight? Next thing, you won't be seeing me at all! Guess our relationship is over."

- Come on! Going out with her friends doesn't mean she won't have time for him ever again.

5. **The 'This or That' Trap** (False Dichotomy):

- Only two extreme choices. "Either we move in together now, or we break up."

- That's manipulation. There are always other choices and ways to meet both of your wants and needs.

6. **The 'After All I've Done' Guilt Trip** (Guilt-Tripping):

- "After everything I've done for you, you can't do this one thing?"

- You never have to do anything you don't want to do, even if your bae did XYZ for you.

7. **The 'It's Your Fault I'm Mad' Blame Shift** (Victim Blaming):

- Shifting the blame for their wrong actions onto you. "You make me angry because you're always messing up." "It's your fault I'm angry, you shouldn't have worn that dress!" Never true! Their actions, their words, their anger – that's on them.

8. **The 'Never Good Enough'** (Goalpost Move):

- Changing what they want after you've done it. "You got a job, but not the one I wanted." "You won the game, but not fast enough." "You got an A, but you didn't win an award." And so on.

9. **The 'I'm Right Because I'm Right' Circle** (Circular Reasoning Fallacy):

- "I'm right because I say I'm right." Uh, nope. You saying you're right doesn't make you right.

10. **The 'Everyone's Doing It'** (Bandwagon Fallacy):

- "All my friends do that, so you should too." Just because others do it doesn't mean it's the right thing for you to do. Your feelings and opinions matter and should be respected.

11. **The 'I'm Older, So I Know Better'** (Appeal to Authority Fallacy):

- "I'm older, so obviously, I know better about this." Being older does NOT mean they know better or that your opinion doesn't matter.

- It can also come in a sneaky way of showing you someone famous or cool who did what they want you to do and then trying to get you to do the same thing. "Jenny is a famous actress and Jenny did it, so you should too."

Why Knowing This Stuff Matters

Recognizing these 'false truths' is like unlocking a secret level in the game of relationships. It helps you see when someone's trying to play mind games. Remember, in a healthy relationship, it's all about respect, honesty, and understanding – not these sneaky mind tricks.

You've got the power to spot these tricks and call them out. Keep your eyes open and trust your gut. You're smarter than these false truths, and you deserve real, honest love. 🖤

OVERCOMING ' FALSE TRUTHS': YOUR REFLECTIVE EXERCISE

Seeing Through the Fog of Words

Ever had someone say something to you that just felt off? Like, they say something hurtful, but they twist it so it sounds almost true? It's like they're using some weird logic to make you feel bad or doubt yourself. Well, it's time to put on your detective hat and see through these 'false truths.' Let's get started!

Step-by-Step Instructions:

1. **Recall the Experience**: Think back to a recent time when someone said something that left you feeling confused, insulted, or just plain bad about yourself.

2. **Write Down the Words**: Jot down exactly what they said. Try to remember their exact words, no matter how harsh they might seem now.

3. **Their 'Logic'**: What reasons did they give you to back up what they said? Did they try to make it sound like they were just stating facts?

4. **Why You Believed Them**: Reflect on why their words seemed believable at the time. Was it because of who they were or how they said it?

5. **Spot the Fallacies**: Now, put on your critical thinking cap. Can you identify any logical fallacies in their argument? Like, were they making a huge generalization or attacking you instead of the issue?

6. **Another Perspective**: Take a step back and try to see the situation in a new light. Is there a different, more positive way to look at it? Maybe they were projecting their own issues onto you, or maybe they were just plain wrong.

Wrapping Up: Seeing the Truth

By doing this exercise, you're learning to separate hurtful words from reality. You're figuring out how to spot when someone's using twisted logic to bring you down. Remember, just because someone says something doesn't make it true. Trust in your own perception, your own feelings, and your own truth. You got this!

Stay strong, keep questioning, and never forget that your perspec- tive matters. You're more than someone else's words – you're a whole universe of thoughts, feelings, and truths. Keep shining your light!

CYBERBULLYING

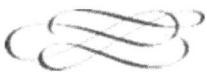

Cyberbullying can totally wreck your self-esteem and make you feel unloved and depressed. If you're being cyberbullied or were cyberbullied, it's important to take care of your mental health. Repeat positive affirmations, do some fun things you love, and spend time in the real world away from the toxicity online.

POSITIVE AFFIRMATIONS TO COMBAT CYBERBULLYING

When you're dealing with cyberbullying, it's super important to remind yourself of your worth. Here are some affirmations to repeat every day. Say them out loud, write them down, or even set them as your phone wallpaper – whatever works for you!

- "I am more than what others say online." "I am worthy of respect and kindness."

- "I am strong and can overcome negativity."

- "My self-worth isn't defined by others' opinions."

- "I choose to focus on the love and support around me."

- "I am capable of rising above hate."

- "My feelings are valid, and I deserve to be heard."

- "I am loved, and I will not let cyberbullying define me."

POSITIVITY EXERCISE: RECL AIMING YOUR SPACE

Step 1: Digital Detox

Start by taking a little break from social media. It's like hitting the pause button on all that negativity. Use this time to do things that make you feel good – reading, hanging out with friends, drawing, dancing – anything that brings you joy.

Step 2: Gratitude Journaling

Every day, write down three things you're grateful for in your life. It could be anything – your pet, your favorite song, a good laugh with a friend. This helps shift your focus from the negative to the positive.

Step 3: Connect with Supporters

Spend time with people who uplift you. Chat with friends who make you laugh or hang out with family who have your back. It's all about surrounding yourself with positivity.

Step 4: Reflect and Grow

At the end of each day, take a few minutes to reflect on something positive that happened or something you did well. It's about recog- nizing the good in every day, no matter how small.

Wrapping Up: You're Stronger Than You Know

Remember, cyberbullying can be tough, but you're tougher. These affirmations and exercises are tools to help you rebuild your confi- dence and keep your head held high. You're amazing, and don't let anyone – especially some online bully – make you think otherwise. 🚀🩶

If you need help, go to Cyberbullying.org for advice and support, and talk to an adult you can trust.

PHYSICAL ABUSE

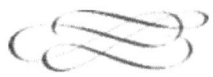

Physical abuse is terribly harmful. One of the most important things to address is the feeling victims have that it's all their

fault and they somehow deserved it.

Even if you weren't physically abused, but if you were abused in any other way, the following exercises will help you overcome the misplaced deep feeling of guilt and shame.

" IT' S YOUR FAULT I HURT YOU! YOU MADE ME DO IT!"

When They Say It's Your Fault – It's Not!

Ever played a game where you get blamed for stuff that's totally out of your control? Like another character shoots at you, or you fall into a trap that the game developer made, and someone's like, "That's totally your fault! You deserved it!" Crazy, right? Well, that's exactly what happens in some relationships when it comes to reacting to stuff.

In an abusive relationship, your partner might hurt you and then say things like, "You made me do it!" or "If only you hadn't said that, I wouldn't have gotten so mad."

You might feel it's unfair but feel guilty and ashamed anyway.

But here's the thing – *it's never your fault. No one deserves to be hurt, EVER.*

Why It's Not Your Fault:

1. **Choice and Control**: Remember, everyone has a choice in how they react. One person might react in a cool, calm way. Another might react violently. If someone chooses to hurt you, it's on them, not you. Just like in a game, if someone shoots at you, it's their decision, not your fault.

2. **Blame Game**: Abusers often play the blame game to control and manipulate you. It's their way of avoiding responsibility for their actions. It's like a magician using misdirection – they want you to look away from what's really happening.

3. **Understanding the Damage**: Being constantly blamed can mess with your head. It can make you doubt yourself and even believe you're the problem. But that's the abuser's voice in your head, not the truth. It's like wearing glasses with the wrong prescription – it distorts your view of reality.

The Psychology Behind It

1. **Gaslighting**: This is when someone tries to make you doubt your own experiences and perceptions. Imagine if someone kept changing the rules of a game but insisted they were always the same. Confusing, right?

2. **Self-Doubt**: Constant blame can lead to self-doubt. It's like if you kept losing in a game and started to think maybe you're just bad at it, even if the game was rigged against you.

3. **Fear and Control**: Abusers use blame to create fear and maintain control. It's their way of keeping you in the game, even when it's harming you.

Breaking Free from Blame

1. **Affirm Your Reality**: Keep a journal or talk to trusted friends about what's happening. It's like keeping a scorecard – it helps you see the game for what it really is.

2. **Seek Support**: Talk to someone who understands, like a counselor or a support group. It's like getting a guide for a really tough game.

3. **Affirmations**: Practice telling yourself the truth – that you're worthy, you're capable, and you don't deserve to be treated badly. It's like giving yourself a pep talk before a big game.

4. **Understand Your Worth**: Remember, you're valuable and deserving of respect. Just like in a game, you're the main character in your life – don't let someone else control your story.

Conclusion: Your Strength and Your Future

Realizing and accepting that the abuse and the blame aren't your fault is like leveling up in understanding yourself. It takes strength, but you've got it. You have the power to step out of the horror game and into a new reality where you're respected, loved, and safe.

Remember, in the story of your life, you're the hero – and heroes deserve happy endings.

DIFFERENT REACTIONS: IT' S ALL ABOUT CHOICES

Picture this: Your friend totally bombs a test. Here's how different peeps might react:

1. **Healthy Reaction**: One friend goes, "Bummer, man. Let's study together next time." That's a chill, supportive vibe.

2. **Unhealthy Reaction**: Her boyfriend flips out, "Bitch, you're so dumb! You're a total loser!" And he slaps her. That's just harsh, abusive, and totally not cool.

Or imagine you're rocking a new outfit that you think is fire, but your BF/GF isn't into it. Check out these reactions:

1. **Healthy Reaction**: They might be like, "Not my style, but you do you!"

2. See, that's respecting your choice.

3. **Unhealthy Reaction**: Or they go all, "You can't wear that! Change now! Or I'll punch you!" That's controlling, abusive, and a major red flag.

Freedom to Choose = Responsibility

Everyone's got the freedom to choose how they react. If your BF/GF chooses to get angry or upset over small stuff or even big stuff – that's on them, not you.

Like, say you can't hang out 'cause you gotta study or chill with your squad.

Here's how it can go down:

1. **Healthy Reaction**: They're like, "Cool, catch you later!" That's understanding and respecting your space.

2. **Unhealthy Reaction**: But if they throw a fit, like "You never spend time with me!" – that's manipulative.

3. Or worse, they punch you or kick you and then say it's your fault because you wanted to hang with your friends. That's abusive and toxic!

The Bottom Line: Their Reaction, Their Responsibility

So here's the deal: how someone reacts is their choice, and it says more about them than about you. If they choose to be under- standing and cool, that's awesome. But if they choose to be controlling or mean, that's on them, and it's not cool.

It's like in a game – if you make a move and someone else freaks out, it's their issue, not yours. You're not responsible for how they choose to react.

Remember, in a healthy relationship, peeps respect each other's choices and reactions. It's about supporting, not controlling. So, next time someone tries to blame you for their reaction, remember, it's their choice, and you don't have to own it. Stay true to you, and don't let anyone mess with your vibe!

WHY IT'S NOT YOUR FAULT

When someone decides to hurt you, it's on them, not you. Let's break it down, teen style:

1. Agency and Choice

Everyone's got their own mind, right? We all make choices based on what we think and believe. So, when someone chooses to hurt you, that's all on them. It's like choosing between a chocolate or vanilla ice cream – it's their pick, based on their taste (or, in this case, their character).

2. Cause and Effect Misinterpretation

Ever been told, "You made me do it"? Nah, that's not how it works. Just because you disagreed or asked a question doesn't mean you caused their hurtful behavior. Their reaction (like getting mad or violent) comes from their own issues, not because of what you did or said.

3. Stimulus and Response

Picture this: You say you like a different band than your friend does. That's the stimulus. If they start yelling at you, that's their choice of response. A chill person might just say, "Cool, different tastes."

The way they respond says a lot about them, not about the band or you.

Everyone reacts differently to a stimulus (like you stating you like Taylor Swift while they like Lady Gaga). You are never responsible for their reaction; therefore, their reaction is not your fault.

Understanding Behavior and Character

1. Behavior Reflects the Person

Ever notice how some people are always chill while others lose their cool over small stuff? That's because people's actions show who they are inside. If someone's always aggressive or mean, it's more about their own issues and less about the people they're mean to.

2. Blame-Shifting: Their Defense Mechanism

When someone's like, "You made me do this," they're actually trying to dodge facing their own problems. It's easier for them to point fingers at you than to admit they've got stuff to work on.

3. Healthy vs. Unhealthy Reactions

Here's the thing: Different people react differently to the same stuff. If one person gets violent over a disagreement while another person stays cool, it shows who they are, not what the disagree- ment was about. It's like two gamers playing the same tough level – one might rage-quit, and the other keeps trying calmly. The game's the same; the players are different.

It's Their Character, Not Your Fault So, bottom line: When someone hurts you, remember that it's their choice and a reflec- tion of who they are. You're not to blame for their actions, and you definitely don't deserve to be treated badly. Stay true to yourself, and don't let anyone's bad vibes change who you are. You're awesome just the way you are!

1. Personal Boundaries

You know how in video games, every character has their own space, their own moves? That's like personal boundaries in real life. You're in charge of your space – your actions, your feelings. But here's the deal: you can't control how others play their game. If someone decides to go rogue, that's on them, not you. Your job? Just keep playing your game the best you can.

2. Self-Compassion

Imagine giving yourself a high-five or a hug every day. That's self- compassion. It's about being your own BFF, understanding that you're not the one messing up when someone else is being mean or hurtful. You deserve to be treated with respect and kindness, no matter what. So next time you're feeling down, remember to treat yourself like you would your best friend.

3. Seeking Healthy Relationships

Let's talk healthy relationships. They're like a perfect playlist – every song complements the other, no track trying to overpower the rest. In a healthy relationship, it's cool to have different opin- ions, and it doesn't turn into a big drama. It's about mutual respect, where both of you get to be your awesome selves without fear of being put down.

So, you like TayTay while he likes Lady Gaga? That's fine! No need to get angry or violent about that.

Wrapping it Up

Understanding all this stuff is kinda like leveling up in life. It's realizing that if someone chooses to be hurtful, it's a reflection of them, not you. You've got to remember, you're not the game controller for someone else's actions. This understanding is huge – it's the start of healing, seeing yourself in a new light, and moving towards the kind of relationship where you're treated like the rockstar you are. Remember, you're awesome just the way you are, and no one has the right to make you feel otherwise!

REFLECTIVE EXERCISES:

The Tale of Two Dogs and a Girl Named Anna

Imagine this: There are two dogs. One's a Rottweiler, a tough- looking dude who's had it rough. He's from a shelter, and in his past life, he was beaten up. Like, whenever his old owner raised a hand, it wasn't for pets, but for hits, especially on his head. Not cool, right?

Then, there's this brown poodle, the chill type. He comes from a super peaceful home where he was treated like a king. Lots of head pats, cuddles, and no shouting or hitting. He's totally into getting his head pet.

So, here comes Anna, this young girl who loves dogs. She goes to pet the Rottweiler, right? But the moment she reaches out, the guy freaks and bites her hand. Ouch!

Next up, Anna tries petting the poodle. And guess what? He's all about it. He licks her hand, wags his tail, and is just living for those head pats.

The Big Questions

Now, think about it: Why did these two dogs react so differently? Anna's the same person with both. She's just being herself, but each dog gives her a totally different reaction.

Is it something Anna did? Or is it more about how each dog's been treated in the past, shaping how they react now?

Do their reactions say anything about Anna being a good or bad person?

And hey, what about the Rottweiler biting Anna? Is that on her? Is she a bad person because he reacted that way?

Or is the bite more about the Rottweiler's past and his choice to react that way?

Write your answers:

_____

_____

_____

_____

_____

Reflecting on the Story

The truth is, it's not Anna's fault the Rottweiler bit her. It was his choice and his action. That's totally on him, it's his fault.

This story is like a mirror, showing us how past experiences shape reactions.

It's a reminder that sometimes, how someone reacts to us has more to do with their past and less with what we're doing in the present.

So, what do you think about Anna's situation?

Remember, like with Anna and the dogs, how people react to us can be about their history, their fears, and their choices. It's not always about what we did or didn't do. Understanding this can help us see things from a different angle and be more empathetic to others and to ourselves. Stay thoughtful, and keep an open heart!

The Tale of Two Step-Brothers and a Puppy

Picture this: Two step-brothers, Ron and Joe. They're like night and day. Ron's got this aggressive, angry vibe. Joe, on the other hand, is chill, kind, and all about spreading love.

Their dad brings home this adorable puppy, Roofus. He's all wiggly, happy, and loves to play. When Roofus wants attention, he does what pups do best – he barks!

Different Reactions to the Same Bark

So, here's the deal. When Roofus barks at Ron, especially when Ron's trying to focus on homework, Ron flips out. He's like, "Bad dog! Be quiet! You're messing up my study time!" Ron sees the barking as a huge no-no. He gets super mad and even hits Roofus.

But check out how Joe handles it. When Roofus barks at him, even if Joe's super busy with homework, he's all calm and understand- ing. He's like, "Not now, Roofus, I gotta study, buddy. Shhh!" If Roofus keeps it up, Joe might toss him a toy or give him a quick

pat before getting back to his books. Joe never gets mad at Roofus. He's all about the cuddles and love.

Thinking Cap Time: Why the Difference?

So, why do Ron and Joe react so differently to the same thing – Roofus barking? Is it because they're just wired differently, each with their own way of dealing with stuff? Or did Roofus somehow make them act like this?

Your Answer: _____

And how about this: Ron says it's Roofus's fault he hit him.

But could Roofus really make Ron and Joe behave so differently? Who's actually responsible for how Ron and Joe react – and why? Your Answer: _____

Now, who 'made' Ron be harsh with Roofus, and who 'made' Joe treat Roofus kindly?

If you think no one 'made' them act that way, why do you think they did what they did?

Your Answer: _____

Wrapping Up: Understanding Reactions

This story shows us that how people react to the same situation can be totally different. It's about their character, their mindset, and their choice – not about the puppy's actions. Remember, just like Ron and Joe, people choose their reactions, and it's not the puppy's (or anyone else's) fault. 🐾

The truth is, even though Ron said, "I hit him because he made me! It's his fault! He barked," it isn't Roofus's fault. It's Ron's choice of how to react to that behavior of barking.

No one can control anyone else's actions. Roofus didn't "make him do it."

Ron behaved that way because he chose to, just like Joe chose to behave in a kind way. It's not Roofus's fault.

In the same way, no matter what 'wrong' thing you may have done, if someone is mean to you, that's their choice, and it's never your fault. There are many other ways to handle a mistake or a 'wrong action,' just like Joe did! It doesn't have to be mean, violent, or hurtful. Remember, everyone makes mistakes, and that's not a sin.

You deserve to be treated with respect, kindness, and love – always.

Affirm: *How someone behaves is their choice, not my fault. I am only responsible for my own actions, and others are only responsible for theirs.*

JOURNALING EXERCISE: TACKLING SELF-BL AME LIKE A BOSS

Hey there! It's time to dive into some real talk with yourself. Grab your journal, find a comfy spot, and let's get those thoughts flow- ing. These questions are all about helping you see things clearer and ditch any unnecessary self-blame. Ready? Let's roll!

1. **Reacting to Your Actions: Think Squad Style:** Ever noticed how different your friends, relations, or adults react differently to the same stuff you do?

Like, one friend laughs off a silly mistake, but another might get all moody about it. One relation is cool about something you did, while the other thinks it's terrible. Reflect on this: when you had a disagreement or goofed up, how did different people react?

Write down their different responses from positive to negative.

Why did each of them react differently? Mention their personali- ties beneath their reactions.

2. **Choices, Choices – It's All You:** Remember a time when you had to respond to someone else's drama or actions? Did you weigh your options on how to react? What made you decide how to respond?

This is about getting how we all have choices, including those peeps who might be blaming you for their stuff.

3. **Spot the Blame Game:** Ever been blamed for someone else losing their cool or doing something wrong? Look back at that. Could they have reacted another way? What would've been a more chill and positive reaction from them?

4. **You're Not the Puppet Master:** Think about a time you felt like it was your fault someone else acted badly. Were you really pulling their strings? If you had a magical remote control for their actions, how would you have made them act? This is about seeing the difference between feeling like it's your fault and actually control- ling someone else's moves.

5. **Controlling Their Reactions – Myth or Reality?** Think about it: if you really could control their reactions, could you make them do silly stuff like singing a love song or dancing on one foot right now? If you can't make them do these things, it means you don't control their actions, not even the hurtful ones. What does this say about the idea that you're responsible for their behavior?

6. **Emotional Influence Check:** Remember a time when you reacted intensely to something someone did. What were you feeling at that moment? How did your emotions steer your reac- tion? This might give you a clue about how others react based on their feelings, not because of what you do.

7. **Journey of Personal Growth:** How have you changed in dealing with conflicts or disagreements? What influenced these changes in you? Think about this: if your responses have evolved, doesn't it show that how we act is a choice shaped by our growth and who we are as people?

8. **Spotting a Healthy Relationship:** Reflect on the healthiest rela- tionship you've seen or been a part of. How are disagreements handled there? What does this tell you about the importance of respect and understanding?

9. **Dealing with False Accusations:** Think back to a time when someone blamed you for something you didn't do. Did their words change the actual truth of the situation?

10. **Why the Blame Game?** Ever wonder why some peeps are quick to point fingers instead of owning up to their stuff? Think about why it's easier for some to blame others than to take respon- sibility. Getting this can be a game-changer in shaking off any blame they try to stick on you.

11. **Rewind and Reframe:** Remember a time when someone tried to make their bad choices your fault? Now, with all you know about personal responsibility, how would you see that situation differently? It's like editing a movie scene with new insights, giving it a whole new meaning.

As you write, remember, the goal is to realize that everyone's responsible for their own actions. You're not to blame for how someone chooses to react, even if they try to make you think so. These prompts are here to help you see that, so take your time, think it through, and let's start turning those pages to a new chapter of understanding and self-compassion.

By working through these questions, you're doing some serious mental muscle-building. You're responsible for your actions, sure, but you can't control others. And hey, that's totally okay. So, keep on journaling, keep on reflecting, and watch yourself grow stronger each day!

AFFIRMATIONS FOR STRENGTH AND RESILIENCE

You've been through a lot, and I want you to know something important – you're stronger and more awesome than you realize.

These affirmations are like little power-ups for your soul. They're here to help you find your inner strength, love yourself more, and build up that resilience that's already inside you. Let's dive into them!

1. **"I am strong, capable, and resilient."** – This is like your personal strength anthem. Say it loud, say it proud. You've got this incredible inner power, and it's time to own it.

2. **"My body is beautiful, and I love it just the way it is."** – Your body has been your buddy through thick and thin. It's time to give it some love and appreciation.

3. **"I forgive myself and accept my feelings."** – Everyone makes mistakes, and that's okay. Forgive yourself like you would forgive your best friend. Your feelings? They're totally valid, no matter what.

4. **"It wasn't my fault."** – Seriously, what happened to you was not your fault. You didn't deserve it, and you're not to blame.

5. **"I have the right to control my body and my life."** – Your body, your rules. Your life, your choices. You're the boss here.

6. **"I am worthy of love, respect, and kindness."** – Yes, you! You deserve all the good things, all the love, all the respect. Don't let anyone tell you otherwise.

7. **"I have the right to be happy."** – Happiness isn't just for others; it's for you too. You deserve to laugh, smile, and have awesome times.

8. **"I deserve safety and peace."** – Feeling safe and at peace is your right. You should feel secure in your world.

9. **"I can create a happy, fulfilling life."** – Your life's story is yours to write, and it can be full of joy, success, and all the things you dream of.

Making Affirmations Part of Your Day

Okay, so why are these affirmations a big deal? They're like daily reminders that help you heal, grow, and find your way back to feeling good about yourself. When you repeat these affirmations, you're slowly rewiring your brain to believe in your awesomeness.

How to Practice Them:

- Stick them on your mirror, so they're the first thing you see in the morning.

- Make them your phone wallpaper.

- Write them in your journal or say them out loud as part of your morning routine.

Remember, healing is a journey, and it's different for everyone. But each time you say these affirmations, you're taking one more step towards feeling stronger, more confident, and totally in charge of your life. Keep going, you're doing amazing!

SEXUAL ABUSE

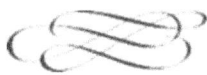

Sexual abuse is very serious. Remember to get help from a professional. EFT can greatly help with sexual trauma.

Affirmations can also help but shouldn't be the only thing you rely on for healing.

AFFIRMATIONS FOR EMOTIONAL HEALING

Here are some affirmations to help with healing and self- acceptance:

1. **"My body is mine, and it's amazing."** Remind yourself that your body is your own, and it deserves love and respect.

2. **"I release guilt and shame. They do not belong to me. I am a good, lovable person, no matter what anyone else did to me. I release all shame now."** Let go of any feelings of guilt or shame. They're not yours to carry; they belong to the one who did it to you.

3. **"I am more than what happened to me."** Your experiences don't define your entire being. You're so much more.

4. **"I am worthy of love and respect, always."** No matter what, you deserve to be treated with kindness and respect.

5. **"My feelings are valid and important."** Your emotions matter. It's okay to feel them fully.

6. **"I am strong and resilient."** You've got a strength inside you that's incredible.

7. **"I have the right to be happy and safe."** You deserve a life filled with happiness and safety.

8. **"I am in charge of my life and my choices."** Remember, you have the power to make decisions for yourself.

9. **"I am healing, one day at a time."** Healing is a journey, and it's okay to take it one step at a time.

10. **"I am enough, just as I am."** You don't need to be anything more than what you are right now.

11. **"My past does not determine my future."** You have the power to shape a different, brighter future.

12. **"Every day, I grow stronger and more confident."** With each day, you're becoming even more amazing.

Remember to say these to yourself, write them down, or even say them out loud. Affirmations can be powerful tools in your journey to healing and self-love. 🖤

SELF-EMPOWERMENT & SELF- ESTEEM

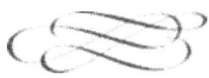

Here are some really helpful affirmations to release unfair guilt, shame, blame, and to amp up your self-confidence.

AFFIRMATIONS TO RELEASE SELF-BL AME AND PAIN

If you've been hurt by someone and then told it's your fault, know that it's NOT true. It's unfair blame.

It's crucial to realize that the responsibility for someone's actions lies solely with them, not with those they affect. These affirma- tions are here to help you release the blame that was wrongfully placed on your shoulders. Repeat each out loud at least 10 times:

1. "Their response is their choice. If they choose an abusive response, that's their choice and not my fault."

2. "There are always many other ways to respond to a situation, including good, kind, calm, peaceful ways."

3. "I am only in control of my own reactions, not anyone else's."

4. "I am not responsible for the actions or mistakes of others. My worth is inherent and independent of their behavior."

5. "I recognize that my past does not define my future. I am capable of creating a life filled with love and respect."

6. "I am worthy of kindness and compassion. My experiences do not diminish my value as a person."

7. "I forgive myself for the times I believed it was my fault. I now know I was doing my best in a difficult situation."

8. "I deserve to be treated with respect and understanding. My feelings and experiences are valid."

9. "I acknowledge that I am only in control of my own actions and responses, not those of others. Their choices reflect on them, not on me."

10. "When someone chooses to hurt me, it is a reflection of their character, not mine. I am not to blame for their decisions."

11. "I release the burden of others' actions. Their behavior is their responsibility, not mine."

12. "The voices that blamed me were wrong. I now choose to listen to my own voice, one that speaks truth and kindness."

13. "I am strong enough to recognize that another's hurtful behavior is a choice they make, and it is never a reflection of my worth."

14. "I trust in my ability to discern right from wrong. Others' attempts to shift blame do not change the truth."

15. "I am free from the falsehood that I am responsible for someone else's actions. I own my story, not their choices."

16. "I am empowered by the knowledge that I cannot control others, only how I respond and grow from my experiences."

17. "I choose to surround myself with people who acknowledge their actions and respect my boundaries. I deserve healthy relationships."

18. "Every day, I grow stronger in the belief that I am not at fault for the harmful choices of others. This truth sets me free."

These affirmations are designed to help you reinforce your under- standing of personal boundaries and responsibility. Remember, healing from such experiences is a journey, and it's okay to take your time to internalize these truths. You're doing wonderfully by seeking out and using these affirmations. Keep nurturing your inner strength and wisdom.

AFFIRMATIONS FOR SELF-EMPOWERMENT

Here's a list of empowering affirmations to help reclaim your power, your life, and the control of your future:

1. "I am the architect of my life; I build its foundation and choose its contents."

2. "I am in control of my life. I can create any life and future I want. I am now creating a happy, successful, fun life."

3. "Every day, I am growing stronger and more empowered."

4. "I possess the qualities needed to be extremely successful and happy."

5. "My ability to conquer challenges is limitless; my potential to succeed is infinite."

6. "I am in control of my narrative and my life's direction."

7. "I am courageous and stand up for myself and my dreams."

8. "Today, I am brimming with energy and overflowing with joy."

9. "My thoughts are filled with positivity, and my life is plentiful with prosperity."

10. "I am my own superhero. I have the power to create change."

11. "I wake up today with strength in my heart and clarity in my mind."

12. "My fears of tomorrow are simply melting away. I own my future."

13. "I am capable of achieving greatness, and I start that journey today."

14. "Every challenge I face is an opportunity to grow and improve."

15. "I am deserving of my dreams, and I reach for them with confidence."

16. "My voice is important, and my opinions matter."

17. "I am surrounded by abundance and seize the opportunities it brings."

18. "I am a unique individual with so much to offer the world."

19. "I choose to focus on what I can control and let go of the rest."

20. "I am a powerful creator. I create the life I want and enjoy it every day."

Remember, repeating these affirmations regularly can profoundly impact your mindset, empowering you to take charge of your life and embrace the future with confidence and strength.

UNPACKING THE FORGIVENESS KIT

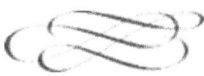

Hey, I totally get it, forgiveness can be super tough, especially if you're still dealing with all those rough emotions. Here's a tip: try EFT (Emotional Freedom Techniques) first to work through the pain and trauma. It's kinda like clearing the clutter before you start redecorating your room. Once the hurt starts to fade, forgiving becomes way easier.

Now, let's talk about some easy forgiveness exercises. These are like your tools for fixing up your emotional space, helping you let go of all that heavy resentment. This way, you can step into a brighter future filled with peace, happiness, and loads of love for the awesome new peeps you're gonna meet and hang with. 💔🌈

1. WRITE A LETTER TO YOURSELF

Here's a simple way to start: Write a letter to yourself. Yep, you heard it right. Pour out all the forgiveness and understanding you can muster. It might feel odd at first, like talking to your reflection, but it's super powerful.

2. POSITIVE MIRRORING

Okay, so here's a super cool trick to help you believe in yourself more, especially if you're feeling down about something personal. It's called Positive Mirroring, and it's kinda like being a cheer- leader for someone else, which in turn helps you too. Here's how it works:

Imagine you're feeling down about something, like maybe you think you're not lovable because of your weight. What you do is to find a picture online of someone who's kinda in the same boat as you. Then, even if you're just chilling alone in your room, start talking out loud to that picture as if you're talking to a real person. Say stuff like, "Hey, you are totally worthy of love just the way you are! Your size? It doesn't define your worth at all!"

Now, here's where the magic happens. The more you keep saying these awesome, positive things to this imaginary person, the more your own brain starts to believe that they're true for you too. You might be wondering, how on earth does that work? Let me explain.

So, imagine inside your brain, there's this little dude who's like a fact checker. His job is to keep all your beliefs in check. The thing is, sometimes he gets it totally wrong, especially if he's holding onto negative untrue stuff like "I'm not worthy of love."

This fact checker is super stubborn and clings to these wrong 'facts,' always finding fake 'proof' to support them. He's like a little warrior, sword in hand, ready to fight off any new ideas that chal- lenge these beliefs.

Now, if you try to hit him with direct affirmations like "I am worthy of love," you're basically picking a fight with him. And let me tell you, it can be tough because this fact checker doesn't back down easily.

But here's a sneaky trick – if you use Positive Mirroring, like telling an imaginary person, "You are worthy of love," you're basi- cally sneaking past this fact checker. He's so busy looking out for direct attacks, he doesn't notice these sneaky side moves. It's like dodging past a security guard while he's busy looking the other way.

By doing this, you're slipping these positive beliefs into your 'brain-computer' without setting off any alarms. And the coolest part? After you do this a bunch of times, your brain starts to actu- ally believe these new, positive things about yourself. It's like updating your brain's software with the best, most positive beliefs. And before you know it, you'll totally believe in your own awesomeness!

So, by doing this Positive Mirroring, you're not only spreading positivity, but you're also rewiring your own brain to believe in your own worth and awesomeness. And that, my friend, is a total win-win!

3. TURN YOUR ABUSER INTO THE VICTIM

Okay, so here's a different way to look at things, especially if you're dealing with all the hurt from an abuser. It's called Positive Projection. It's like flipping the script in your mind and seeing things from a whole new angle. Picture this: your abuser, instead of being this big, scary figure, is actually a victim too. Sounds wild, right? But stick with me here.

A lot of times, people who hurt others have been hurt in the same way themselves. It's like a messed-up cycle. So, the trick to breaking free from all that emotional chaos they caused you is to see them as a victim. Not in a way where you feel sorry for them or anything, but in a way that lets you say, "Okay, I'm done being hurt by you."

Here's how you can do it: First, write down all the nasty stuff your abuser made you feel. Stuff like, "It's my fault they treated me badly; I don't deserve to be treated kindly," or, "My thoughts don't matter."

Then flip it around and write down the total opposite, but in a positive way. Think, "It was never my fault they were mean. I deserve kindness. My thoughts are important."

Now, imagine saying all these positive things *to your abuser*. I know, sounds super weird, right? But as you do this, you start seeing them in a different light. You might even begin to realize that they were acting out because of their own deep issues. Like, maybe they were super pushy about their music taste because they were never allowed to enjoy their own tunes growing up. Or maybe they felt ugly because their dad insulted them, so they kept picking on you and making you feel unattractive.

The wild part is, as you keep doing this, you'll start feeling free from all that pain.

It will crumble away. The crushing pain on your heart will begin to lift and vanish. The burning knots of anger in your stomach will cool off and disappear.

Plus, you'll begin to believe all those good things about *yourself!* It's like breaking a weird dark curse, you know? You might not know everything about your abuser's past, but by flipping the script and seeing them as a victim, you release yourself from their hold in a really weird but effective way.

And that's the real magic – you start healing and believing in your own awesomeness.

4. FORGIVENESS AFFIRMATIONS

Repeat affirmations to forgive yourself and the abuser.

Affirmations for Self-Forgiveness:

1. "I forgive myself and let go of all guilt and shame. I did my best in that moment with what I knew."

2. "I acknowledge that I handled the situation the best way I could at the time. I forgive myself completely."

3. "I release myself from the burden of past mistakes. I was doing my best to survive and navigate."

4. "I understand that everyone makes mistakes, including me. I forgive myself and embrace learning from my past."

5. "I choose to be kind to myself about the past. I did what I thought was right then, and now I know more."

6. "I let go of self-blame. My past actions don't define my worth or my future."

7. "I forgive myself for not leaving sooner. I understand that my fear and uncertainty were real and valid."

8. "I free myself from the weight of what I 'should' have done. I'm focusing on what I can do now."

9. "I am more than my past experiences. I forgive myself and grow stronger each day."

10. "Every day, I choose self-forgiveness and self-compassion. I am healing and learning."

11. "I forgive myself and release all guilt and shame now. I did what I could at the time with the knowledge I had. I did my best, and that's enough. I was just doing what I could to handle a difficult situation. I forgive myself. I let it all go now."

Affirmations for Forgiving the Abuser and Letting Go:

1. "I choose to forgive, not for them, but for my peace of mind. I release the hold this pain has on me."

2. "I let go of anger and resentment. Holding onto these feelings only hurts me."

3. "Forgiving doesn't mean forgetting. It means freeing myself from the chains of bitterness."

4. "I forgive as an act of strength, not because what happened was okay, but because I choose to free myself from their hold over my life. I am taking back my power and peace."

5. "Forgiving is my way of saying I am no longer your victim. It does not condone your actions but releases me from the pain they caused. My forgiveness is my path to a life where you no longer have any power to hurt me."

6. "I forgive, understanding that it's a step towards my own healing and freedom."

7. "I release the power that this hurt has over my life. I choose peace and healing."

8. "I acknowledge that forgiving is for me. It's my path to emotional freedom and closure."

9. "I understand that forgiveness is a process, and I am patient with myself as I journey through it."

10. "I forgive, not because it's easy, but because I deserve to move on and live a life filled with joy."

11. "By forgiving, I reclaim my power and my peace. I am not defined by what happened to me."

12. "I let go of the past hurt and embrace a future filled with hope and healing."

Remember, these affirmations are tools to guide you on your journey of healing and self-compassion. They are like small, daily steps towards a more peaceful and empowered you.

PASSING THE TORCH OF HOPE

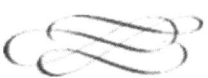

You've journeyed through the pages, discovered secrets to escape toxic chains, and now you're standing in the light of newfound wisdom. It's your turn to be the beacon for others who are still navigating through the darkness.

By sharing your genuine thoughts about this book on Amazon, you're not just leaving a review; you're guiding lost souls to a safe harbor. Your words can be a signpost for fellow teens searching for a way out of the shadows of harmful relationships.

Your support means the world. It's how we spread the message of hope and healing far and wide. By passing on your insights, you're contributing to a safer, kinder world for teens everywhere.

Thank you for being an integral part of this mission. With each person you reach, you're helping to strengthen the chain of posi- tive change.

Together, we're not just reading about change; we're making it happen.

Jordan Phoenix

Click here to share your journey and light the way for others on Amazon.

LEAVE A REVIEW!

CONCLUSION

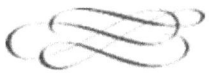

As we wrap up this bonus Self-Help Guide, I want to leave you with some heartfelt wishes and reminders. You've got an array of tools at your fingertips to continue healing and to protect yourself from future harm. Therapy offers professional guidance and support. Affirmations help reinforce positive self-beliefs. Talking to an AI chatbot like 'Hope' gives you a safe space to express your- self and seek advice, any time you need it. EFT/Tapping is a powerful technique for releasing emotional pain. Journaling lets you reflect deeply on your thoughts and feelings. And critical thinking helps you question and understand your experiences more clearly.

Remember, every step you take is a step towards a brighter, more empowered future. You've got the strength, the tools, and the resilience not just to heal but to thrive. Wishing you all the happi- ness and health as you continue on your incredible journey. You've got this!

REFERENCES

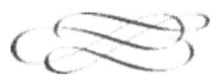

Agaron, S. (2021, April 16). *Mood Meter: identify and regulate your emotions*. Brain Street. https://shamay.com/mood-meter-app-review/

Aravind, V., Krishnaram, V., & Thasneem, Z. (2012). *Boundary Crossings and Violations in Clinical Settings. Indian Journal of Psychological Medicine, 34*(1), 21– 24. https://doi.org/10.4103/0253-7176.96151

Breaking the Cycle: How to Heal Unhealthy Teenage Relationships. (2023, July 25). ThreePeaks Ascent Residential Treatment Center. https://threepeakstreat ment.com/residential-treatment-for-teens/unhealthy-relationships/

Chaturvedi, S. K. (2023). The Good, Bad and not so Bad of Positive Thinking and Recovery. *Journal of Psychosocial Rehabilitation and Mental Health, 10*(2), 129–130. https://doi.org/10.1007/s40737-023-00348-1

Counseling, S. C. (2023, July 20). *9 Ways to Rebuild Self-Esteem After a Toxic Relationship*. Seattle Christian Counseling. https://seattlechristiancounseling. com/articles/9-ways-to-rebuild-self-esteem-after-a-toxic-relationship

Creswell, J. D., Dutcher, J. M., Klein, W. M. P., Harris, P. R., & Levine, J. M. (2013). *Self-Affirmation Improves Problem-Solving under Stress. PLoS ONE, 8*(5), e62593. https://doi.org/10.1371/journal.pone.0062593

15 Tips for Letting Go of a Relationship That Is Not Healthy - GoodTherapy.org Therapy Blog. (2023, November 10). GoodTherapy.org Therapy Blog. https://www. goodtherapy.org/blog/15-tips-for-letting-go-of-a-relationship-that-is-not- healthy-0829167/

15 Tips to Build Self Esteem and Confidence in Teens. (n.d.). Big Life Journal. https:// biglifejournal.com/blogs/blog/build-self-esteem-confidence-teens

Gordon, S. (2021, July 26). *What Teens Need to Know About Boundaries.* Verywell Family. https://www.verywellfamily.com/boundaries-what-every-teen-needs- to-know-5119428

Gordon, S. (2022, September 29). *Benefits of Mindfulness for Kids and Teens.* Verywell Family. https://www.verywellfamily.com/benefits-of-mindfulness- for-kids-4769017

How do I heal from a toxic relationship as a teenager? (n.d.). Quora. https://www. quora.com/How-do-I-heal-from-a-toxic-relationship-as-a-teenager-2

Kassel, G. (2023, December 7). *9 Signs You're Dating a Narcissist — and How to Get Out.* Healthline. https://www.healthline.com/health/mental-health/am-i- dating-a-narcissist

K. (2023, August 18). *20 Simple Ways How to Self-Love After Toxic Relationship.* Pinch of Attitude. https://www.pinchofattitude.com/self-love-after-toxic- relationship/

K. (2023, July 20). *Online Teen Safety Guide.* StaySafe.org. https://staysafe.org/ teens/

Lonczak, H. S. (2023, October 9). *What Is Gaslighting? 20 Techniques to Stop Emotional Abuse.* PositivePsychology.com. https://positivepsychology.com/ gaslighting-emotional-abuse/

Love is Respect. (2018, September 10). *loveisrespect.org.* Loveisrespect.org. https:// www.loveisrespect.org/

L. (2023, September 4). *Importance of a support system after a toxic relationship - Recovery from Toxic Relationships.* Recovery From Toxic Relationships. https:// toxicrelationshiprecovery.com/importance-of-a-support-system-after-a-toxic- relationship/

Resilience. (n.d.). https://www.apa.org. https://www.apa.org/topics/resilience

Self-esteem and teenagers - ReachOut Parents. (n.d.). https://parents.au.reachout.com/ common-concerns/everyday-issues/self-esteem-and-teenagers

Smith, M. (2024, February 5). *Setting Healthy Boundaries in Relationships.* HelpGuide.org. https://www.helpguide.org/articles/relationships-communica tion/setting-healthy-boundaries-in-relationships.htm

Social Media and Teen Romantic Relationships. (2019, December 31). Pew Research Center: Internet, Science & Tech. https://www.pewresearch.org/internet/ 2015/10/01/social-media-and-romantic-relationships/

Sun, H., Yuan, C., Qian, Q., Shu-Zhi, H., & Luo, Q. (2022, March 31). *Digital Resilience Among Individuals in School Education Settings: A Concept Analysis Based on a Scoping Review.* Frontiers in Psychiatry. https://doi.org/10.3389/fpsyt. 2022.858515

Surviving A Relationship Break-Up -Top 20 Strategies. (n.d.). https://www.mcgill.ca/ counselling/files/counselling/surviving_a_break-up_-_20_strategies_0.pdf Sweeney, E. (n.d.). *Toxic Relationships and Teenage Mental Health.* The BHS Beat.

https://bhsbeat.org/3124/student-life/toxic-relationships-and-teenage- mental-health/

Teens and social media use: What's the impact? (2024, January 18). Mayo Clinic. https://www.mayoclinic.org/healthy-lifestyle/tween-and-teen-health/in- depth/teens-and-social-media-use/art-20474437

Tips for Building Healthy Relationships with Your Teenagers. (n.d.). CAMH. https:// www.camh.ca/en/health-info/guides-and-publications/tips-for-building- healthy-relationships-with-your-teenagers

Treatment, A. A. (2023, March 14). *Why Healthy Boundaries Are So Important in*

Recovery. Ashley Addiction Treatment. https://www.ashleytreatment.org/ rehab-blog/boundaries-in-recovery/